THE BLOOD TYPE O DIET COOKBOOK

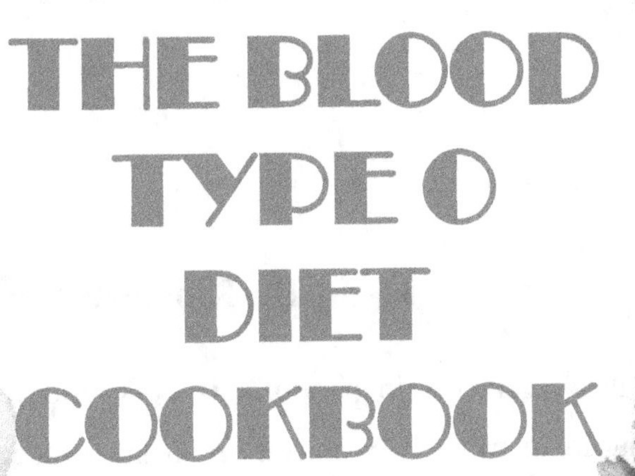

Dr. Kimberly Carlos

Copyright © 2024 by Dr. Kimberly Carlos

All rights reserved. No part of this publication may be reproduced, distributed, or transmitted in any form or by any means, including photocopying, recording, or other electronic or mechanical methods, without the prior written permission of the publisher, except in the case of brief quotations embodied in critical reviews and certain other noncommercial uses permitted by copyright law.

TABLE OF CONTENT

GOOD HEALTH IS FAR BETTER THAN WEALTH...

INTRODUCTION

The Blood Type O Diet is a nutritional approach that tailors dietary recommendations based on an individual's blood type.

According to the Blood Type Diet theory, each blood type (O, A, B, and AB) is associated with specific ancestral diets, and following the appropriate diet for your blood type can optimize health and well-being.

Benefits of the Blood Type O Diet:

1. Improved Digestion and Nutrient Absorption: The Blood Type O Diet suggests that certain foods may be better tolerated by individuals with blood type O, leading to enhanced digestion and nutrient absorption.

2. Weight Management: Advocates of the Blood Type O Diet claim that following the recommended diet can support weight management by aligning with the specific needs of blood type O individuals.

3. Enhanced Energy Levels: The tailored food choices are believed to provide sustainable energy for individuals with blood type O, potentially reducing feelings of fatigue.

4. Optimized Metabolism: The diet emphasizes foods that may support the metabolism of blood type O individuals, aiding in efficient calorie utilization and overall metabolic health.

Key Principles of the Blood Type O Diet:

1. High-Protein Emphasis: The Blood Type O Diet recommends a focus on lean, high-quality proteins such as meat, fish, and poultry, reflecting the supposed ancestral diet of early hunter-gatherers with blood type O.

2. Limited Grains and Legumes: Grains and legumes, particularly those containing lectins, are advised to be consumed in moderation or avoided to support digestive health.

3. Emphasis on Vegetables: Non-starchy vegetables are encouraged as a rich source of vitamins, minerals, and antioxidants, promoting overall health.

4. Moderate Fruit Intake: While fruits are included, there may be specific recommendations to prioritize certain fruits over others, taking into account individual blood type characteristics.

Personalizing Nutrition for Optimal Health

The Blood Type O Diet is a personalized approach to nutrition, emphasizing the unique dietary needs of individuals with blood type O. While the scientific evidence supporting the Blood Type Diet is limited, some individuals report positive outcomes. As with any dietary plan, it's essential to consult with healthcare professionals and consider personal preferences and nutritional requirements.

Embarking on the Blood Type O Diet can be an intriguing journey into understanding the potential impact of blood type on dietary needs. By incorporating the principles of this diet, individuals may discover a way of eating that aligns with their body's unique characteristics and contributes to overall health and vitality.

How to Adopt a Blood Type O Diet Plan

Adopting a Blood Type O Diet plan involves making specific food choices that align with the principles of the Blood Type Diet, which suggests that individuals with blood type O thrive on certain types of foods. Here's a guide on how to adopt a Blood Type O Diet:

1. Know Your Blood Type:

Before adopting the Blood Type O Diet, it's crucial to confirm your blood type through a blood test. Knowing your blood type is the foundation for tailoring your diet to your specific needs.

2. Understand the Blood Type O Diet Guidelines:

Familiarize yourself with the general guidelines of the Blood Type O Diet. These guidelines typically include recommendations for protein sources, carbohydrates, fruits, and vegetables that are believed to be beneficial or avoided for individuals with blood type O.

3. Focus on High-Quality Proteins:

The Blood Type O Diet emphasizes the consumption of lean, high-quality proteins, such as meat, fish, and poultry. Incorporate these protein sources into your meals to support muscle development and energy.

4. Limit Grains and Legumes:

Reduce or eliminate the intake of grains and legumes, as they may contain lectins that could potentially be less compatible with blood type O individuals. Opt for alternative carbohydrate sources such as sweet potatoes and quinoa.

5. Prioritize Vegetables:

Non-starchy vegetables are a key component of the Blood Type O Diet. Include a variety of vegetables in your meals to ensure a rich supply of essential vitamins, minerals, and antioxidants.

6. Moderate Fruit Consumption:

While fruits are generally recommended, there may be specific fruits that are considered more beneficial for individuals with blood type O. Moderation is key, and it's advisable to choose fruits that align with the diet guidelines.

7. Incorporate Beneficial Supplements:

Some versions of the Blood Type O Diet recommend specific supplements to address potential nutrient deficiencies. Consult with a healthcare professional to determine if supplements are necessary for your individual needs.

8. Stay Hydrated:

Adequate hydration is essential for overall health. Drink plenty of water throughout the day to support digestion and other bodily functions.

9. Listen to Your Body:

Pay attention to how your body responds to different foods. Individual variations exist, and it's essential to adjust the diet based on personal preferences, tolerances, and any potential health concerns.

10. Consult with a Professional:

Before making significant changes to your diet, especially based on specific blood type recommendations, consult with a healthcare professional or a registered dietitian. They can provide personalized guidance based on your overall health and specific needs.

Adopting a Blood Type O Diet involves a thoughtful and informed approach to nutrition. While the scientific evidence supporting the Blood Type Diet is limited, some individuals find success in following these guidelines. Remember that dietary choices are personal, and it's essential.

DELICIOUS BLOOD TYPE O DIET RECIPES

1. Grilled Turkey and Vegetable Skewers

Ingredients:

- 1 pound turkey breast, cut into chunks

- 1 zucchini, sliced

- 1 red bell pepper, cut into chunks

- 1 red onion, cut into chunks

- 2 tablespoons olive oil

- 2 tablespoons lemon juice

- 2 garlic cloves, minced

- 1 teaspoon dried oregano

- Salt and pepper to taste

Instructions:

1. In a bowl, mix olive oil, lemon juice, minced garlic, dried oregano, salt, and pepper to create a marinade.

2. Place turkey chunks in the marinade, ensuring they are well-coated. Let it marinate in the refrigerator for at least 30 minutes.

3. Preheat the grill to medium-high heat.

4. Thread marinated turkey chunks, zucchini slices, red bell pepper chunks, and red onion chunks onto skewers.

5. Grill the skewers for about 10-15 minutes, turning occasionally until the turkey is cooked through and the vegetables are slightly charred.

6. Serve the skewers with a side of steamed quinoa or a leafy green salad.

2. Quinoa and Vegetable Stir-Fry

Ingredients:

- 1 cup quinoa, rinsed

- 2 cups water or vegetable broth

- 2 tablespoons olive oil

- 1 cup broccoli florets

- 1 cup sliced carrots

- 1 cup sliced mushrooms

- 1 cup snow peas, ends trimmed

- 2 garlic cloves, minced

- 2 tablespoons tamari or soy sauce

- 1 teaspoon sesame oil

- 1 teaspoon grated ginger

- Sesame seeds for garnish (optional)

Instructions:

1. In a saucepan, combine quinoa and water or vegetable broth. Bring to a boil, then reduce heat, cover, and simmer for 15-20 minutes or until quinoa is cooked and water is absorbed.

2. In a large pan or wok, heat olive oil over medium-high heat.

3. Add minced garlic and grated ginger, sautéing for about 30 seconds until fragrant.

4. Add broccoli, carrots, mushrooms, and snow peas to the pan. Stir-fry the vegetables for 5-7 minutes until they are tender-crisp.

5. Pour tamari or soy sauce and sesame oil over the vegetables, stirring to coat evenly.

6. Add the cooked quinoa to the pan and toss everything together until well combined.

7. Garnish with sesame seeds if desired and serve hot.

3. Baked Salmon with Lemon and Dill

Ingredients:

- 4 salmon fillets

- 2 tablespoons olive oil

- 2 tablespoons fresh lemon juice

- 1 teaspoon dried dill

- 2 cloves garlic, minced

- Salt and pepper to taste

- Lemon slices for garnish

Instructions:

1. Preheat the oven to 400°F (200°C).

2. Place salmon fillets on a baking sheet lined with parchment paper.

3. In a small bowl, mix olive oil, lemon juice, dried dill, minced garlic, salt, and pepper.

4. Brush the salmon fillets with the lemon and dill mixture, ensuring they are well-coated.

5. Bake for 15-20 minutes or until the salmon is cooked through and flakes easily with a fork.

6. Garnish with lemon slices before serving.

4. Turkey and Vegetable Lettuce Wraps

Ingredients:

- 1 pound ground turkey

- 1 tablespoon olive oil

- 1 onion, finely chopped

- 2 bell peppers (any color), diced

- 1 zucchini, diced

- 2 cloves garlic, minced

- 2 tablespoons tamari or soy sauce

- 1 teaspoon ground ginger

- Iceberg lettuce leaves for wrapping

Instructions:

1. In a skillet, heat olive oil over medium heat. Add chopped onion and cook until softened.

2. Add ground turkey to the skillet, breaking it apart with a spoon and cooking until browned.

3. Add diced bell peppers, zucchini, and minced garlic to the skillet. Cook for an additional 5-7 minutes until vegetables are tender.

4. Stir in tamari or soy sauce and ground ginger. Mix well and let it cook for an additional 2-3 minutes.

5. Spoon the turkey and vegetable mixture into individual iceberg lettuce leaves, creating wraps.

6. Serve immediately, and you can drizzle additional tamari or soy sauce if desired.

5. Quinoa Stuffed Bell Peppers

Ingredients:

- 4 bell peppers, halved and seeds removed

- 1 cup quinoa, cooked

- 1 can (15 oz) black beans, drained and rinsed

- 1 cup corn kernels (fresh or frozen)

- 1 cup diced tomatoes

- 1 cup diced avocado

- 1/4 cup fresh cilantro, chopped

- 1 teaspoon ground cumin

- Salt and pepper to taste

Instructions:

1. Preheat the oven to 375°F (190°C).

2. In a large bowl, combine cooked quinoa, black beans,

corn, diced tomatoes, diced avocado, cilantro, ground cumin, salt, and pepper.

3. Place bell pepper halves in a baking dish and stuff each half with the quinoa mixture.

4. Cover the baking dish with foil and bake for 25-30 minutes, or until the peppers are tender.

5. Garnish with additional cilantro before serving.

6. Grilled Chicken Salad with Balsamic Vinaigrette

Ingredients:

- 2 boneless, skinless chicken breasts

- 1 tablespoon olive oil

- Salt and pepper to taste

- Mixed salad greens (spinach, arugula, and romaine)

- Cherry tomatoes, halved

- Cucumber, sliced

- Red onion, thinly sliced

- Feta cheese, crumbled (optional)

 Balsamic Vinaigrette:

- 3 tablespoons balsamic vinegar

- 1/4 cup extra-virgin olive oil

- 1 teaspoon Dijon mustard

- 1 clove garlic, minced

- Salt and pepper to taste

Instructions:

1. Preheat the grill or grill pan.

2. Brush chicken breasts with olive oil and season with salt and pepper.

3. Grill the chicken for 6-8 minutes per side or until fully cooked.

4. In a large bowl, combine salad greens, cherry tomatoes, cucumber, and red onion.

5. Slice grilled chicken and place it on top of the salad.

6. In a small bowl, whisk together balsamic vinegar, olive oil, Dijon mustard, minced garlic, salt, and pepper to make the vinaigrette.

7. Drizzle the vinaigrette over the salad and toss gently. Top with crumbled feta if desired.

7. Lentil and Vegetable Soup

Ingredients:

- 1 cup green or brown lentils, rinsed

- 1 onion, chopped

- 2 carrots, diced

- 2 celery stalks, diced

- 3 cloves garlic, minced

- 1 can (14 oz) diced tomatoes

- 6 cups vegetable broth

- 1 teaspoon ground cumin

- 1 teaspoon paprika

- 1/2 teaspoon thyme

- Salt and pepper to taste

- Fresh parsley, chopped (for garnish)

Instructions:

1. In a large pot, sauté chopped onion, carrots, celery, and garlic until softened.

2. Add lentils, diced tomatoes, vegetable broth, cumin, paprika, thyme, salt, and pepper to the pot. Stir well.

3. Bring the soup to a boil, then reduce heat and let it simmer for 25-30 minutes or until lentils are tender.

4. Adjust seasoning if needed.

5. Ladle the soup into bowls, garnish with fresh parsley, and serve.

8. Stir-Fried Shrimp with Vegetables

Ingredients:

- 1 pound shrimp, peeled and deveined

- 2 tablespoons tamari sauce (gluten-free soy sauce)

- 1 tablespoon olive oil

- 1 bell pepper, sliced

- 1 zucchini, sliced

- 1 cup broccoli florets

- 2 cloves garlic, minced

- 1 tablespoon ginger, grated

- 2 green onions, sliced

- Sesame seeds for garnish

Instructions:

1. In a bowl, marinate shrimp in tamari sauce for about 15 minutes.

2. Heat olive oil in a wok or large skillet over medium-high heat.

3. Add garlic and ginger, sauté for 1-2 minutes until fragrant.

4. Add marinated shrimp and cook until pink and opaque, about 2-3 minutes.

5. Add bell pepper, zucchini, and broccoli. Stir-fry for an additional 3-4 minutes until vegetables are tender-crisp.

6. Garnish with sliced green onions and sesame seeds before serving.

9. Quinoa and Vegetable Stuffed Peppers

Ingredients:

- 4 large bell peppers, halved and seeds removed

- 1 cup quinoa, cooked

- 1 can (15 oz) black beans, drained and rinsed

- 1 cup corn kernels (fresh or frozen)

- 1 cup cherry tomatoes, halved

- 1 avocado, diced

- 1/4 cup fresh cilantro, chopped

- Juice of 1 lime

- Salt and pepper to taste

Instructions:

1. Preheat the oven to 375°F (190°C).

2. In a large bowl, combine cooked quinoa, black beans, corn, cherry tomatoes, avocado, cilantro, lime juice, salt, and pepper.

3. Stuff each bell pepper half with the quinoa mixture.

4. Place stuffed peppers in a baking dish and cover with foil.

5. Bake for 25-30 minutes until peppers are tender.

6. Serve with additional lime wedges and cilantro if desired.

10. Grilled Portobello Mushrooms with Balsamic Glaze

Ingredients:

- 4 large portobello mushrooms, stems removed

- 2 tablespoons balsamic vinegar

- 2 tablespoons olive oil

- 2 cloves garlic, minced

- 1 teaspoon dried thyme

- Salt and pepper to taste

- Fresh parsley for garnish

Instructions:

1. Preheat the grill or grill pan.

2. In a bowl, whisk together balsamic vinegar, olive oil, minced garlic, dried thyme, salt, and pepper.

3. Brush both sides of each portobello mushroom with the balsamic mixture.

4. Grill mushrooms for 4-5 minutes per side until tender.

5. Garnish with fresh parsley before serving.

11. Lentil and Vegetable Soup

Ingredients:

- 1 cup green or brown lentils, rinsed

- 1 onion, chopped

- 2 carrots, diced

- 2 celery stalks, diced

- 3 cloves garlic, minced

- 1 can (14 oz) diced tomatoes

- 6 cups vegetable broth

- 1 teaspoon dried thyme

- 1 teaspoon cumin

- Salt and pepper to taste

- Olive oil for sautéing

Instructions:

1. In a large pot, heat olive oil over medium heat. Sauté onions, carrots, and celery until softened.

2. Add minced garlic and continue sautéing for 1-2 minutes.

3. Pour in vegetable broth, lentils, diced tomatoes, thyme, cumin, salt, and pepper.

4. Bring to a boil, then reduce heat and simmer for 25-30 minutes or until lentils are tender.

5. Adjust seasoning as needed before serving.

12. Turkey and Vegetable Skewers

Ingredients:

- 1 pound turkey breast, cut into chunks

- 1 red onion, cut into wedges

- 1 bell pepper, cut into squares

- 1 zucchini, sliced

- 2 tablespoons olive oil

- 2 tablespoons tamari sauce (gluten-free soy sauce)

- 1 teaspoon smoked paprika

- 1 teaspoon dried oregano

- Wooden skewers, soaked in water

Instructions:

1. Preheat the grill or grill pan.

2. In a bowl, mix olive oil, tamari sauce, smoked paprika, and dried oregano to create a marinade.

3. Thread turkey chunks, red onion wedges, bell pepper squares, and zucchini slices onto the soaked skewers.

4. Brush the skewers with the marinade.

5. Grill for 8-10 minutes, turning occasionally, until the turkey is cooked through and vegetables are tender.

6. Serve the skewers with a side of quinoa or a green salad.

13. Quinoa and Black Bean Salad

Ingredients:

- 1 cup cooked quinoa

- 1 can (15 oz) black beans, drained and rinsed

- 1 cup cherry tomatoes, halved

- 1 cucumber, diced

- 1/4 cup red onion, finely chopped

- 1/4 cup fresh cilantro, chopped

- Juice of 1 lime

- 2 tablespoons olive oil

- Salt and pepper to taste

Instructions:

1. In a large bowl, combine cooked quinoa, black beans, cherry tomatoes, cucumber, red onion, and cilantro.

2. In a small bowl, whisk together lime juice, olive oil, salt, and pepper.

3. Pour the dressing over the quinoa mixture and toss until well combined.

4. Chill in the refrigerator for at least 30 minutes before serving.

14. Baked Salmon with Lemon and Dill

Ingredients:

- 4 salmon fillets

- 2 tablespoons olive oil

- 1 lemon, sliced

- 2 tablespoons fresh dill, chopped

- Salt and pepper to taste

Instructions:

1. Preheat the oven to 400°F (200°C).

2. Place salmon fillets on a baking sheet lined with parchment paper.

3. Drizzle olive oil over the salmon and season with salt and pepper.

4. Top each fillet with lemon slices and sprinkle fresh dill over the top.

5. Bake for 15-20 minutes or until the salmon flakes easily with a fork.

6. Serve with a side of steamed asparagus or your favorite vegetables.

15. Berry and Spinach Smoothie

Ingredients:

- 1 cup fresh spinach

- 1/2 cup blueberries

- 1/2 cup strawberries, hulled

- 1 banana

- 1 cup almond milk

- 1 tablespoon chia seeds

- Ice cubes (optional)

Instructions:

1. In a blender, combine spinach, blueberries, strawberries, banana, almond milk, and chia seeds.

2. Blend until smooth and creamy.

3. Add ice cubes if desired and blend again.

4. Pour into a glass and enjoy this refreshing and nutrient-packed smoothie.

Certainly! Here are two more Blood Type O-friendly recipes:

16. Grilled Chicken and Vegetable Skewers

Ingredients:

- 1 pound chicken breast, cut into cubes

- 1 zucchini, sliced

- 1 red bell pepper, cut into chunks

- 1 yellow bell pepper, cut into chunks

- 1 red onion, cut into wedges

- 2 tablespoons olive oil

- 2 cloves garlic, minced

- 1 teaspoon dried oregano

- Salt and pepper to taste

Instructions:

1. In a bowl, mix olive oil, minced garlic, dried oregano, salt, and pepper to create a marinade.

2. Thread chicken cubes and vegetable pieces onto skewers.

3. Brush the skewers with the marinade, ensuring even coating.

4. Preheat the grill to medium-high heat.

5. Grill the skewers for 10-15 minutes, turning occasionally,

until the chicken is fully cooked and vegetables are tender.

6. Serve with a side of quinoa or brown rice.

17. Lentil and Vegetable Stir-Fry

Ingredients:

- 1 cup green or brown lentils, cooked

- 1 broccoli crown, florets separated

- 1 carrot, julienned

- 1 bell pepper (any color), thinly sliced

- 1 cup snap peas, ends trimmed

- 2 tablespoons soy sauce (low sodium)

- 1 tablespoon sesame oil

- 1 teaspoon grated ginger

- 2 cloves garlic, minced

- 1 green onion, sliced

- Sesame seeds for garnish

Instructions:

1. In a wok or large skillet, heat sesame oil over medium-high heat.

2. Add ginger and garlic, sauté for 1-2 minutes until fragrant.

3. Add broccoli, carrot, bell pepper, and snap peas. Stir-fry for 5-7 minutes until vegetables are tender yet crisp.

4. Add cooked lentils to the vegetables.

5. Pour soy sauce over the mixture and toss until well coated.

6. Cook for an additional 2-3 minutes.

7. Garnish with sliced green onions and sesame seeds before serving.

18. Turkey and Sweet Potato Hash

Ingredients:

- 1 pound ground turkey

- 2 sweet potatoes, peeled and diced

- 1 red onion, chopped

- 2 cloves garlic, minced

- 1 teaspoon smoked paprika

- 1 teaspoon dried thyme

- Salt and pepper to taste

- Fresh parsley for garnish

Instructions:

1. In a large skillet, brown ground turkey over medium heat until cooked through.

2. Add diced sweet potatoes, chopped red onion, and minced garlic to the skillet.

3. Season with smoked paprika, dried thyme, salt, and pepper.

4. Cook, stirring occasionally, until sweet potatoes are tender.

5. Garnish with fresh parsley before serving.

20. Grilled Salmon with Lemon and Dill

Ingredients:

- 4 salmon fillets

- 2 lemons, thinly sliced

- 2 tablespoons olive oil

- 2 tablespoons fresh dill, chopped

- Salt and pepper to taste

Instructions:

1. Preheat the grill to medium-high heat.

2. Rub salmon fillets with olive oil and season with salt and pepper.

3. Place lemon slices on top of each fillet and sprinkle with fresh dill.

4. Grill for 4-5 minutes per side or until salmon is cooked to your liking.

5. Serve with a side of steamed asparagus or a green salad.

21. Quinoa and Vegetable Stuffed Bell Peppers

Ingredients:

- 4 large bell peppers, halved and seeds removed

- 1 cup quinoa, cooked

- 1 can black beans, drained and rinsed

- 1 cup corn kernels (fresh or frozen)

- 1 cup cherry tomatoes, halved

- 1 cup spinach, chopped

- 1 teaspoon cumin

- 1 teaspoon chili powder

- Salt and pepper to taste

- Shredded cheddar cheese (optional)

Instructions:

1. Preheat the oven to 375°F (190°C).

2. In a large bowl, combine cooked quinoa, black beans, corn, cherry tomatoes, and spinach.

3. Season with cumin, chili powder, salt, and pepper. Mix well.

4. Spoon the mixture into halved bell peppers.

5. If desired, sprinkle shredded cheddar cheese on top.

6. Bake for 25-30 minutes or until the peppers are tender.

7. Serve with a dollop of Greek yogurt or avocado slices.

22. Stir-Fried Beef and Broccoli

Ingredients:

- 1 pound flank steak, thinly sliced

- 2 cups broccoli florets

- 1 red bell pepper, thinly sliced

- 3 cloves garlic, minced

- 2 tablespoons coconut aminos

- 1 tablespoon olive oil

- 1 teaspoon arrowroot powder (or cornstarch)

- Salt and pepper to taste

- Sesame seeds for garnish

Instructions:

1. In a bowl, mix sliced flank steak with arrowroot powder, salt, and pepper.

2. Heat olive oil in a wok or skillet over medium-high heat.

3. Add minced garlic and sliced steak, stir-frying until the meat is browned.

4. Toss in broccoli florets and sliced red bell pepper, continuing to stir-fry until vegetables are tender yet crisp.

5. Pour coconut aminos over the mixture, ensuring even coating.

6. Cook for an additional 2-3 minutes until everything is well combined and heated through.

7. Garnish with sesame seeds before serving.

23. Lentil and Vegetable Soup

Ingredients:

- 1 cup green or brown lentils, rinsed

- 1 onion, diced

- 2 carrots, diced

- 2 celery stalks, diced

- 3 cloves garlic, minced

- 1 can diced tomatoes

- 6 cups vegetable broth

- 1 teaspoon dried thyme

- 1 teaspoon ground cumin

- Salt and pepper to taste

- Fresh parsley for garnish

Instructions:

1. In a large pot, sauté diced onion, carrots, celery, and garlic until softened.

2. Add lentils, diced tomatoes, vegetable broth, thyme, cumin, salt, and pepper to the pot.

3. Bring the mixture to a boil, then reduce the heat and let it

simmer for 25-30 minutes or until lentils are tender.

4. Adjust seasonings if needed.

5. Ladle the soup into bowls and garnish with fresh parsley before serving.

24. Grilled Salmon with Lemon and Dill

Ingredients:

- 4 salmon fillets

- 1 lemon, sliced

- 2 tablespoons olive oil

- 1 tablespoon fresh dill, chopped

- 2 cloves garlic, minced

- Salt and pepper to taste

Instructions:

1. Preheat the grill to medium-high heat.

2. In a small bowl, mix olive oil, minced garlic, chopped dill, salt, and pepper to create a marinade.

3. Place salmon fillets on a plate and brush them with the marinade.

4. Top each fillet with lemon slices.

5. Grill the salmon for about 4-5 minutes per side or until it easily flakes with a fork.

6. Serve with additional lemon slices and a sprinkle of fresh dill.

25. Quinoa and Vegetable Stir-Fry

Ingredients:

- 1 cup quinoa, cooked

- 1 cup broccoli florets

- 1 bell pepper, thinly sliced

- 1 zucchini, sliced

- 1 carrot, julienned

- 2 tablespoons tamari (gluten-free soy sauce)

- 1 tablespoon sesame oil

- 1 teaspoon ginger, grated

- 2 green onions, chopped

- Sesame seeds for garnish

Instructions:

1. In a large skillet or wok, heat sesame oil over medium-high heat.

2. Add broccoli, bell pepper, zucchini, and carrot, stir-frying until vegetables are tender-crisp.

3. Stir in cooked quinoa, tamari, and grated ginger, mixing well.

4. Cook for an additional 2-3 minutes to heat through.

5. Garnish with chopped green onions and sesame seeds before serving.

26. Turkey and Sweet Potato Skillet

Ingredients:

- 1 lb ground turkey

- 2 sweet potatoes, peeled and diced

- 1 onion, diced

- 2 cloves garlic, minced

- 1 tablespoon olive oil

- 1 teaspoon smoked paprika

- Salt and pepper to taste

- Fresh parsley for garnish

Instructions:

1. In a large skillet, heat olive oil over medium heat.

2. Add diced sweet potatoes and cook until they begin to soften.

3. Add ground turkey, breaking it apart with a spatula and cook until browned.

4. Stir in diced onion and minced garlic, cooking until the onion is translucent.

5. Season with smoked paprika, salt, and pepper.

6. Cook until sweet potatoes are tender and turkey is cooked through.

7. Garnish with fresh parsley before serving.

27. Stir-Fried Bok Choy with Ginger and Garlic

Ingredients:

- 1 bunch bok choy, chopped

- 2 tablespoons coconut oil

- 1 tablespoon fresh ginger, grated

- 2 cloves garlic, minced

- 1 tablespoon tamari (gluten-free soy sauce)

- Sesame seeds for garnish

Instructions:

1. Heat coconut oil in a wok or skillet over medium-high heat.

2. Add grated ginger and minced garlic, sautéing for 1-2 minutes.

3. Add chopped bok choy and stir-fry until leaves are wilted and stems are tender-crisp.

4. Drizzle tamari over the bok choy and toss to coat evenly.

5. Garnish with sesame seeds before serving.

28. Berry and Spinach Salad

Ingredients:

- 2 cups baby spinach

- 1 cup mixed berries (strawberries, blueberries, raspberries)

- 1/4 cup walnuts, chopped

- 2 tablespoons balsamic vinaigrette dressing

- Feta cheese crumbles (optional)

Instructions:

1. In a large bowl, combine baby spinach, mixed berries, and chopped walnuts.

2. Drizzle balsamic vinaigrette dressing over the salad and toss to coat.

3. If desired, sprinkle feta cheese crumbles on top.

4. Serve immediately and enjoy this refreshing salad.

29. Grilled Salmon with Lemon and Rosemary

Ingredients:

- 2 salmon fillets

- 1 lemon, sliced

- 2 tablespoons olive oil

- 2 cloves garlic, minced

- 1 tablespoon fresh rosemary, chopped

- Salt and pepper to taste

Instructions:

1. Preheat the grill to medium-high heat.

2. In a small bowl, mix olive oil, minced garlic, chopped rosemary, salt, and pepper.

3. Brush the salmon fillets with the olive oil mixture.

4. Place lemon slices on top of each fillet.

5. Grill the salmon for 4-5 minutes per side or until cooked to your liking.

6. Serve with additional lemon wedges and a side of steamed vegetables.

30. Quinoa and Vegetable Stir-Fry

Ingredients:

- 1 cup quinoa, cooked

- 1 cup broccoli florets

- 1 bell pepper, sliced

- 1 carrot, julienned

- 2 tablespoons tamari (gluten-free soy sauce)

- 1 tablespoon sesame oil

- 2 green onions, chopped

- Sesame seeds for garnish

Instructions:

1. In a large skillet or wok, heat sesame oil over medium-high heat.

2. Add broccoli, bell pepper, and julienned carrot, stirring

frequently.

3. Once the vegetables are tender-crisp, add cooked quinoa to the skillet.

4. Drizzle tamari over the mixture and toss to combine.

5. Stir in chopped green onions and cook for an additional 2 minutes.

6. Garnish with sesame seeds before serving.

31. Turkey and Sweet Potato Hash

Ingredients:

- 1 pound ground turkey

- 2 sweet potatoes, peeled and diced

- 1 onion, finely chopped

- 2 cloves garlic, minced

- 1 teaspoon paprika

- 1 teaspoon dried thyme

- Salt and pepper to taste

- Olive oil for cooking

Instructions:

1. Heat olive oil in a skillet over medium heat.

2. Add chopped onion and minced garlic, sauté until softened.

3. Add ground turkey and cook until browned.

4. Stir in diced sweet potatoes, paprika, dried thyme, salt, and pepper.

5. Cover and cook until sweet potatoes are tender, stirring occasionally.

32. Spinach and Mushroom Salad with Balsamic Vinaigrette

Ingredients:

- 2 cups fresh spinach leaves

- 1 cup sliced mushrooms

- 1/4 cup chopped red onion

- 1/4 cup crumbled feta cheese

- 2 tablespoons balsamic vinegar

- 1 tablespoon olive oil

- 1 teaspoon Dijon mustard

- Salt and pepper to taste

Instructions:

1. In a large bowl, combine spinach, sliced mushrooms, chopped red onion, and feta cheese.

2. In a small bowl, whisk together balsamic vinegar, olive oil, Dijon mustard, salt, and pepper.

3. Drizzle the vinaigrette over the salad and toss gently to coat.

33. Grilled Chicken with Lemon and Herbs

Ingredients:

- 4 boneless, skinless chicken breasts

- Zest and juice of 1 lemon

- 2 tablespoons fresh thyme, chopped

- 1 tablespoon fresh rosemary, chopped

- 2 cloves garlic, minced

- Salt and pepper to taste

- Olive oil for brushing

Instructions:

1. Preheat the grill to medium-high heat.

2. In a small bowl, mix lemon zest, lemon juice, chopped thyme, chopped rosemary, minced garlic, salt, and pepper.

3. Brush the chicken breasts with olive oil and then coat them with the lemon and herb mixture.

4. Grill the chicken for 6-8 minutes per side or until cooked through.

34. Shrimp and Broccoli Stir-Fry

Ingredients:

- 1 pound shrimp, peeled and deveined

- 2 cups broccoli florets

- 1 red bell pepper, sliced

- 2 tablespoons tamari sauce (gluten-free soy sauce)

- 1 tablespoon olive oil

- 2 cloves garlic, minced

- 1 teaspoon grated ginger

- 1 teaspoon sesame oil

- Green onions for garnish

- Sesame seeds for garnish

Instructions:

1. In a wok or large skillet, heat olive oil over medium-high heat.

2. Add minced garlic and grated ginger, stir-fry for 30 seconds.

3. Add shrimp and cook until they turn pink and opaque.

4. Add broccoli and red bell pepper, stir-fry until vegetables are tender-crisp.

5. Pour tamari sauce and sesame oil over the mixture, toss to combine.

6. Garnish with chopped green onions and sesame seeds before serving.

35. Quinoa and Vegetable Stuffed Peppers

Ingredients:

- 4 large bell peppers, halved and seeds removed

- 1 cup quinoa, cooked

- 1 cup black beans, drained and rinsed

- 1 cup corn kernels (fresh or frozen)

- 1 cup cherry tomatoes, halved

- 1/2 cup red onion, finely chopped

- 1/4 cup fresh cilantro, chopped

- 1 teaspoon ground cumin

- 1 teaspoon chili powder

- Salt and pepper to taste

- Olive oil for drizzling

Instructions:

1. Preheat the oven to 375°F (190°C).

2. In a large bowl, combine cooked quinoa, black beans, corn, cherry tomatoes, red onion, cilantro, ground cumin, chili powder, salt, and pepper.

3. Drizzle olive oil over the halved bell peppers and place them in a baking dish.

4. Spoon the quinoa mixture into each pepper half.

5. Cover the baking dish with foil and bake for 25-30 minutes or until peppers are tender.

6. Serve with a side of avocado slices or a dollop of Greek yogurt.

36. Grilled Lemon Herb Chicken

Ingredients:

- 4 boneless, skinless chicken breasts

- 2 lemons, juiced

- 3 tablespoons olive oil

- 2 cloves garlic, minced

- 1 teaspoon dried oregano

- 1 teaspoon dried thyme

- Salt and pepper to taste

- Fresh parsley for garnish

Instructions:

1. In a bowl, mix lemon juice, olive oil, minced garlic, dried oregano, dried thyme, salt, and pepper to create a marinade.

2. Place chicken breasts in a zip-top bag and pour the marinade over them. Seal the bag and refrigerate for at least 30 minutes, allowing the flavors to infuse.

3. Preheat the grill to medium-high heat.

4. Grill the chicken breasts for 6-8 minutes per side or until cooked through.

5. Garnish with fresh parsley before serving.

37. Sweet Potato and Turkey Chili

Ingredients:

- 1 pound ground turkey

- 2 sweet potatoes, peeled and diced

- 1 onion, diced

- 2 cloves garlic, minced

- 1 can (15 oz) diced tomatoes

- 1 can (15 oz) black beans, drained and rinsed

- 1 can (15 oz) kidney beans, drained and rinsed

- 1 cup low-sodium chicken broth

- 2 tablespoons chili powder

- 1 teaspoon ground cumin

- Salt and pepper to taste

- Avocado slices for garnish

Instructions:

1. In a large pot, brown the ground turkey over medium heat.

2. Add diced sweet potatoes, diced onion, and minced garlic. Cook until the onion is softened.

3. Stir in diced tomatoes, black beans, kidney beans, chicken broth, chili powder, ground cumin, salt, and pepper.

4. Bring the mixture to a boil, then reduce the heat and let it simmer for 20-25 minutes or until sweet potatoes are tender.

5. Serve the chili in bowls, garnished with avocado slices.

38. Grilled Salmon with Lemon and Dill

Ingredients:

- 4 salmon fillets

- Juice of 1 lemon

- 2 tablespoons olive oil

- 2 cloves garlic, minced

- 1 tablespoon fresh dill, chopped

- Salt and pepper to taste

- Lemon wedges for serving

Instructions:

1. Preheat the grill to medium-high heat.

2. In a bowl, mix lemon juice, olive oil, minced garlic, chopped dill, salt, and pepper to create a marinade.

3. Place salmon fillets in a shallow dish and pour the marinade over them. Let it marinate for at least 20 minutes.

4. Grill the salmon for about 4-5 minutes per side or until it flakes easily with a fork.

5. Serve with lemon wedges.

39. Quinoa and Vegetable Stir-Fry

Ingredients:

- 1 cup quinoa, cooked

- 1 tablespoon sesame oil

- 1 onion, thinly sliced

- 2 bell peppers (any color), thinly sliced

- 1 zucchini, thinly sliced

- 1 cup broccoli florets

- 2 tablespoons low-sodium soy sauce

- 1 tablespoon rice vinegar

- 1 teaspoon ginger, grated

- 2 cloves garlic, minced

- Green onions for garnish

Instructions:

1. Heat sesame oil in a large skillet over medium-high heat.

2. Add sliced onion, bell peppers, zucchini, and broccoli. Stir-fry for 5-7 minutes or until vegetables are tender-crisp.

3. In a small bowl, mix soy sauce, rice vinegar, grated ginger, and minced garlic.

4. Add cooked quinoa to the skillet and pour the sauce over the quinoa and vegetables. Stir well to combine.

5. Garnish with chopped green onions before serving.

40. Turkey and Vegetable Lettuce Wraps

Ingredients:

- 1 pound ground turkey

- 1 tablespoon olive oil

- 1 onion, diced

- 2 carrots, julienned

- 1 bell pepper (any color), diced

- 3 cloves garlic, minced

- 2 tablespoons low-sodium soy sauce

- 1 tablespoon hoisin sauce

- 1 teaspoon sesame oil

- Iceberg lettuce leaves for wrapping

Instructions:

1. In a large pan, heat olive oil over medium heat. Add ground turkey and cook until browned.

2. Add diced onion, julienned carrots, diced bell pepper, and

minced garlic. Cook until vegetables are tender.

3. In a small bowl, mix soy sauce, hoisin sauce, and sesame oil. Pour the sauce over the turkey and vegetable mixture. Stir to combine.

4. Spoon the mixture onto individual iceberg lettuce leaves, creating wraps.

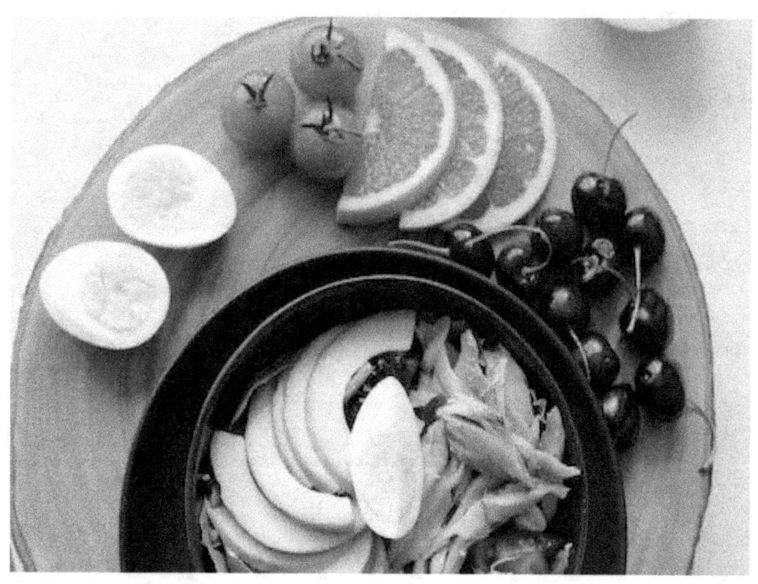

CONCLUSION

The Blood Type O Diet Cookbook is a comprehensive guide that empowers individuals with blood type O to make informed and health-conscious choices in their culinary journey.

By aligning dietary patterns with specific blood types, this cookbook aims to optimize well-being, promote energy, and support overall health.

Through a rich collection of recipes that are not only delicious but also tailored to the unique needs of blood type O individuals, this cookbook becomes a valuable companion on the path to a healthier lifestyle.

As you embark on this nutritional adventure, remember that the journey to well-being is a personalized one. The carefully crafted recipes in this cookbook offer a flavorful array of options, ensuring that adhering to the Blood Type O Diet is both enjoyable and sustainable.

Each dish is designed to not only cater to dietary preferences but also contribute to the overall vitality and vitality of individuals following this specific blood type protocol.

May this cookbook serve as a source of inspiration, guiding you toward mindful and healthful choices in your daily culinary endeavors.

Embrace the flavorful diversity, nourish your body, and savor the satisfaction of eating in harmony with your unique blood type.

Here's to a healthier, happier, and more vibrant you!

www.ingramcontent.com/pod-product-compliance
Lightning Source LLC
Chambersburg PA
CBHW050853260726
48660CB00006B/2614